88 Organic Meal and Juice Recipes for Ovarian Cancer:

The Natural Way to Fight Cancer

By

Joe Correa CSN

COPYRIGHT

© 2017 Live Stronger Faster Inc.

All rights reserved

Reproduction or translation of any part of this work beyond that permitted by section 107 or 108 of the 1976 United States Copyright Act without the permission of the copyright owner is unlawful.

This publication is designed to provide accurate and authoritative information in regard to the subject matter covered. It is sold with the understanding that neither the author nor the publisher is engaged in rendering medical advice. If medical advice or assistance is needed, consult with a doctor. This book is considered a guide and should not be used in any way detrimental to your health. Consult with a physician before starting this nutritional plan to make sure it's right for you.

ACKNOWLEDGEMENTS

This book is dedicated to my friends and family that have had mild or serious illnesses so that you may find a solution and make the necessary changes in your life.

88 Organic Meal and Juice Recipes for Ovarian Cancer:

The Natural Way to Fight Cancer

By

Joe Correa CSN

CONTENTS

Copyright

Acknowledgements

About The Author

Introduction

88 Organic Meal and Juice Recipes for Ovarian Cancer: The Natural Way to Fight Cancer

Additional Titles from This Author

ABOUT THE AUTHOR

After years of Research, I honestly believe in the positive effects that proper nutrition can have over the body and mind. My knowledge and experience has helped me live healthier throughout the years and which I have shared with family and friends. The more you know about eating and drinking healthier, the sooner you will want to change your life and eating habits.

Nutrition is a key part in the process of being healthy and living longer so get started today. The first step is the most important and the most significant.

INTRODUCTION

88 Organic Meal and Juice Recipes for Ovarian Cancer: The Natural Way to Fight Cancer

By Joe Correa CSN

Ovarian cancer is becoming more common every day. Learning to prevent this form of cancer is essential and can be done by consuming the right types of food to allow your body to heal on its own. These meal and juice recipes are based on tasty and healthy ingredients and will strengthen your immune system, restore intestinal integrity, and provide essential nutrients ranging from amino acids to vitamins and minerals.

Today, the popularity of healthy meals and juicing fruits and vegetables is greater than ever before. This positive trend has reminded us of all the health benefits raw foods have. We may or may not have the time to eat healthy, but the fact is that everybody has a couple of minutes to prepare a delicious juice in the morning and start the day in the best possible manner. Returning to these old fashioned healing methods will bring us many benefits.

When we talk about ovarian cancer, the best possible ingredients are avocado, cabbage, bell peppers, tomatoes, asparagus, green tea, grapefruits, ginger, and berries. These powerful ingredients should be the basis of your ovarian cancer-fighting juices.

Juicing is not some new diet trend but a powerful healing tool you can easily implement in your daily routine. By combining great tasting juices with powerful meals, you are creating the ideal environment for ovarian cancer recovery and prevention. If you want to stop ovarian cancer, start eating smarter by using these unique recipes to make a definitive change in your life!

88 ORGANIC MEAL AND JUICE RECIPES FOR OVARIAN CANCER: THE NATURAL WAY TO FIGHT CANCER

1. **Broccoli Cabbage Juice**

Ingredients:

2 cups of broccoli, chopped

1 cup of green cabbage, torn

1 small green apple, cored

1 cup of cauliflower, chopped

2 tbsp of spring onions, chopped

¼ tsp of turmeric, ground

1 oz of water

Preparation:

Wash the broccoli and trim off the outer layers. Chop into small pieces and fill the measuring cup. Reserve the rest for later.

Wash the cabbage thoroughly under cold running water and drain. Torn into small pieces and set aside.

Wash the apple and cut lengthwise in half. Remove the core and cut into bite-sized pieces. Set aside.

Wash the cauliflower and trim off the outer leaves. Chop into small pieces and fill the measuring cup. Reserve the rest in the refrigerator.

Rinse the onion stalk and chop into small pieces. Set aside.

Now, combine broccoli, cabbage, apple, cauliflower, and onions in a juicer and process until juiced.

Transfer to a serving glass and stir in the turmeric and water. Refrigerate for 10 minutes before serving.

Nutritional information per serving: Kcal: 127, Protein: 6.6g, Carbs: 37.9g, Fats: 1.1g

2. Green Tea Juice

Ingredients:

1 tsp of green tea powder

2 cups of spinach, torn

1 cup of watercress, torn

1 cup of kale, torn

1 cup of Swiss chard, torn

¼ tsp of ginger, ground

1 oz of water

Preparation:

Combine, spinach, watercress, kale, and Swiss chard in a large colander. Wash thoroughly under cold running water. Slightly drain and torn into small pieces.

Place the tea powder in a small bowl. Add 3 tbsp of hot water and stir well. Set aside for 3 minutes.

Now, combine spinach, watercress, kale, and Swiss chard in a juicer and process until juiced. Transfer to a serving glass and stir in the ginger and water.

Refrigerate for 20 minutes before serving.

Enjoy!

Nutritional information per serving: Kcal: 87, Protein: 16.3g, Carbs: 22.9g, Fats: 2.4g

3. Asparagus Bell Pepper Juice

Ingredients:

1 cup of asparagus, trimmed

1 large green bell pepper, chopped

1 cup of celery, chopped

¼ tsp of turmeric, ground

¼ tsp of ginger, ground

1 oz of water

Preparation:

Wash the asparagus and trim off the woody ends. Cut into small pieces and fill the measuring cup. Reserve the rest in the refrigerator.

Wash the bell pepper and cut lengthwise in half. Remove the stem and seeds. Chop into small pieces and set aside.

Wash the celery and chop into small pieces. Set aside.

Now, combine asparagus, pepper, and celery in a juicer and process until well juiced. Transfer to a serving glass and stir in the turmeric, ginger, and water.

Add some ice and serve immediately.

Enjoy!

Nutritional information per serving: Kcal: 48, Protein: 5.1g, Carbs: 15.8g, Fats: 0.6g

4. Grapefruit Orange Juice

Ingredients:

1 whole grapefruit, peeled

1 large orange, peeled

1 cup of cucumber, sliced

1 cup of papaya, chopped

¼ tsp of cinnamon, ground

2 tbsp of coconut water

Preparation:

Peel the grapefruit and orange. Divide into wedges. Cut each wedge in half and set aside.

Wash the cucumber and cut into thin slices. Fill the measuring cup and reserve the rest for later.

Peel the papaya and cut into small chunks. Fill the measuring cup and reserve the rest in the refrigerator.

Now, combine grapefruit, orange, cucumber, and papaya in a juicer and process until well juiced.

Transfer to a serving glass and stir in the cinnamon and coconut water.

Refrigerate for 10 minutes before serving.

Nutritional information per serving: Kcal: 214, Protein: 4.6g, Carbs: 65.4g, Fats: 1g

5. Cauliflower Carrot Juice

Ingredients:

1 cup of cauliflower, chopped

2 large carrots, sliced

1 large radish, chopped

1 cup of turnip greens, torn

¼ tsp of ginger, ground

2 oz of water

Preparation:

Trim off the outer leaves of the cauliflower. Wash it and chop into small pieces. Fill the measuring cup and reserve the rest for later.

Wash and peel the carrots. Cut into thin slices and set aside.

Wash the radish and chop into small pieces. Set aside.

Wash the turnip greens thoroughly under cold running water. Drain and torn into small pieces. Set aside.

Now, combine cauliflower, carrots, radish, and turnip greens in a juicer and process until juiced. Transfer to a serving glass and stir in the ginger and water.

Add some ice and serve immediately.

Nutritional information per serving: Kcal: 75, Protein: 4.3g, Carbs: 23.3g, Fats: 0.8g

6.   Pomegranate Banana Juice

Ingredients:

1 cup of pomegranate seeds

1 large banana, chopped

1 small Granny Smith's apple, cored

1 cup of raspberries

¼ tsp of ginger, ground

Preparation:

Cut the top of the pomegranate fruit using a sharp paring knife. Slice down to each of the white membranes inside of the fruit. Pop the seeds into a measuring cup and set aside.

Peel the banana and cut into small pieces. Set aside.

Wash the apple and cut lengthwise in half. Remove the core and cut into bite-sized pieces. Set aside.

Rinse the raspberries under cold running water using a colander. Drain and set aside.

Now, combine pomegranate seeds, banana, apple, and raspberries in a juicer and process until juiced. Transfer to a serving glass and stir in the ginger.

Add some ice and serve immediately.

Nutritional information per serving: Kcal: 265, Protein: 5.1g, Carbs: 81.6g, Fats: 2.5g

7. Artichoke Spinach Juice

Ingredients:

1 large artichoke, chopped

1 cup of fresh spinach, torn

1 cup of green cabbage, torn

1 cup of avocado, cubed

¼ tsp of turmeric, ground

Preparation:

Trim off the outer layers of the artichoke using a sharp paring knife. Cut into bite-sized pieces and set aside.

Combine spinach and cabbage in a large colander. Wash thoroughly under cold running water. Drain and torn into small pieces. Set aside.

Peel the avocado and cut lengthwise in half. Remove the pit and cut into small cubes. Fill the measuring cup and reserve the rest in the refrigerator.

Now, combine artichoke, spinach, cabbage, and avocado in a juicer and process until juiced. Transfer to a serving glass and stir in the turmeric.

Refrigerate for 10 minutes before serving.

Nutritional information per serving: Kcal: 282, Protein: 15.4g, Carbs: 42.6g, Fats: 23.2g

8. Pineapple Blackberry Juice

Ingredients:

1 cup of pineapple, chunked

1 cup of blackberries

1 cup of fresh mint, chopped

1 whole lime, peeled

2 oz of coconut water

Preparation:

Using a sharp paring knife, cut the top of the pineapple. Gently remove all hard skin and slice it into thin slices. Fill the measuring cup and reserve the rest for later.

Place the blackberries in a large colander. Rinse thoroughly under cold running water. Drain and set aside.

Wash the mint and drain. Chop into small pieces and set aside.

Peel the lime and cut lengthwise in half. Set aside.

Now, combine pineapple, blackberries, mint, and lime in a juicer. Process until well juiced and transfer to a serving glass.

Stir in the coconut water and add few ice cubes before serving. Enjoy!

Nutritional information per serving: Kcal: 125, Protein: 4g, Carbs: 42.9g, Fats: 1.2g

9. Pumpkin Chard Juice

Ingredients:

1 cup of pumpkin, chopped

1 cup of Swiss chard, torn

1 medium-sized zucchini, chopped

1 cup of cucumber, sliced

¼ tsp of ginger, ground

1 oz of water

Preparation:

Cut the top of a pumpkin. Cut lengthwise in half and then scrape out the seeds. Cut one large wedge and peel it. Cut into small cubes and fill the measuring cup. Reserve the rest in the refrigerator.

Wash the Swiss chard thoroughly under cold running water. Drain and torn into small pieces. Set aside.

Wash the zucchini and cut into thin slices. Set aside.

Wash the cucumber and cut into slices. Fill the measuring cup and reserve the rest for later.

Now, combine pumpkin, Swiss chard, zucchini, and cucumber in a juicer and process until juiced. Transfer to a serving glass and stir in the ginger and water.

Serve cold.

Nutritional information per serving: Kcal: 65, Protein: 4.5g, Carbs: 16.8g, Fats: 0.8g

10. Lemon Mango Juice

Ingredients:

2 whole lemons, peeled and halved

1 cup of mango, chunked

1 whole grapefruit, peeled and wedged

1 small Granny Smith's apple, cored

¼ tsp of ginger, ground

Preparation:

Peel the lemons and cut each lengthwise in half. Set aside.

Peel the mango and cut into chunks. Fill the measuring cup and reserve the rest for later. Set aside.

Peel the grapefruit and divide into wedges. Cut each wedge in half and set aside.

Wash the apple and cut lengthwise in half. Remove the core and cut into bite-sized pieces. Set aside.

Now, combine lemon, mango, grapefruit, and apple in a juicer and process until juiced. Transfer to a serving glass and stir in the ginger.

Add few ice cubes and serve immediately.

Enjoy!

Nutritional information per serving: Kcal: 65, Protein: 4.5g, Carbs: 16.8g, Fats: 0.8g

11.   Beet-Orange Juice

Ingredients:

1 cup of beets, trimmed and sliced

1 large orange, peeled

1 cup of black grapes

1 whole apricot, pitted

1 tbsp of coconut water

Preparation:

Wash the beets and trim off the green parts. Cut into thin slices and fill the measuring cup. Reserve the rest for later.

Peel the orange and divide into wedges. Cut each wedge in half and set aside.

Rinse the grapes and remove the stems. Set aside.

Wash the apricot and cut lengthwise in half. Remove the pit and cut into small pieces. Set aside.

Now, combine beets, orange, grapes, and apricots in a juicer and process until well juiced. Transfer to a serving glass and stir in the coconut water.

Add some ice and serve immediately.

Nutritional information per serving: Kcal: 184, Protein: 4.9g, Carbs: 54.3g, Fats: 0.9g

12. Cherry Plum Juice

Ingredients:

1 cup of cherries, pitted

2 whole plums, pitted and chopped

1 small green apple, cored

1 cup of strawberries, chopped

1 tbsp of coconut water

¼ tsp of ginger, ground

Preparation:

Wash the cherries thoroughly using a large colander. Drain and cut each in half. Remove the pits and cut into small pieces. Set aside.

Wash the plums and cut in half. Remove the pits and cut into small bite-sized pieces. Set aside.

Wash the apple and cut lengthwise in half. Remove the core and cut into small pieces. Set aside.

Wash the strawberries and remove the stems. Cut into small pieces and fill the measuring cup. Reserve the rest for later. Set aside.

Now, combine cherries, plums, apple, and strawberries in a juicer and process until juiced. Transfer to a serving glass and stir in the coconut water and ginger.

Add some crushed ice and serve immediately.

Nutritional information per serving: Kcal: 236, Protein: 4.2g, Carbs: 70.3g, Fats: 1.3g

13. Pear Cranberry Juice

Ingredients:

1 large pear, chopped

1 cup of cranberries

1 whole lemon, peeled

1 cup of watermelon, chunked

¼ tsp of cinnamon, ground

1 oz of water

Preparation:

Wash the pear and cut in half. Remove the core and cut into small pieces. Set aside.

Place the cranberries in a colander and rinse under cold running water. Drain and set aside.

Peel the lemon and cut lengthwise in half. Set aside.

Cut the watermelon in half. Cut one large wedge and wrap the rest in a plastic foil and refrigerate. Peel the slice and cut into small cubes. Remove the pits and fill the measuring cup. Set aside.

Now, combine pear, cranberries, lemon, and watermelon in a juicer and process until well juiced. Transfer to a serving glass and stir in the cinnamon and water.

Refrigerate for 10 minutes before serving.

Nutritional information per serving: Kcal: 186, Protein: 2.8g, Carbs: 64.1g, Fats: 0.8g

14. Strawberry Avocado Juice

Ingredients:

1 cup of strawberries, chopped

1 cup of avocado, cubed

1 large peach, chopped

1 large Granny Smith's apple, cored

¼ tsp of cinnamon, ground

¼ tsp of ginger, ground

2 tsp of coconut water

Preparation:

Wash the strawberries and remove the stems. Cut into bite-sized pieces and fill the measuring cup. Reserve the rest for later.

Peel the avocado and cut in half. Remove the pit and cut into small cubes. Fill the measuring cup and reserve the rest for later.

Wash the peach and cut lengthwise in half. Remove the pit and cut into bite-sized pieces. Set aside.

Wash the apple and cut in half. Remove the core and chop into small pieces. Set aside.

Now, combine strawberries, avocado, peach, and apple in a juicer and process until juiced. Transfer to a serving glass and stir in the cinnamon, ginger, and coconut water.

Refrigerate for 15 minutes before serving.

Nutritional information per serving: Kcal: 386, Protein: 6.5g, Carbs: 68.6g, Fats: 23.2g

15. Celery Basil Juice

Ingredients:

1 cup of celery, chopped

1 cup of fresh basil, torn

1 cup of cucumber, sliced

1 whole lime, peeled

1 medium-sized apple, cored

Preparation:

Wash the celery and cut into small pieces. Set aside.

Wash the basil thoroughly under cold running water. Drain and torn into small pieces. Set aside.

Wash the cucumber and cut into thin slices. Fill the measuring cup and reserve the rest for later. Set aside.

Peel the lime and cut lengthwise in half. Set aside.

Wash the apple and cut lengthwise in half. Remove the core and cut into bite-sized pieces. Set aside.

Now, combine celery, basil, cucumber, lime, and apple in a juicer and process until well juiced. Transfer to a serving glass and add some crushed ice.

Serve immediately.

Nutritional information per serving: Kcal: 109, Protein: 2.7g, Carbs: 31.9g, Fats: 0.7g

16. Orange Plum Juice

Ingredients:

1 large orange, peeled

1 whole plum, chopped

1 cup of cantaloupe, chopped

1 cup of fresh mint, torn

¼ tsp of turmeric, ground

¼ tsp of ginger, ground

Preparation:

Peel the orange and divide into wedges. Cut each wedge in half and set aside.

Wash the plum and cut in half. Remove the pit and chop into small pieces. Set aside.

Cut the cantaloupe in half. Scoop out the seeds and flesh. Cut and peel one large wedge. Chop into chunks and fill the measuring cup. Reserve the rest of the cantaloupe in a refrigerator.

Wash the mint thoroughly under cold running water. Torn into small pieces and set aside.

Now, combine orange, plum, cantaloupe, and mint in a juicer and process until juiced. Transfer to a serving glass and stir in the turmeric and ginger.

Add some ice and serve immediately.

Enjoy!

Nutritional information per serving: Kcal: 151, Protein: 4.4g, Carbs: 45.6g, Fats: 0.9g

17. Fennel Collard Greens Juice

Ingredients:

1 whole fennel bulb, chopped

1 cup of collard greens, chopped

1 cup of cucumber, sliced

1 whole lemon, peeled

1 oz of water

¼ tsp of cayenne pepper, ground

Preparation:

Trim off the fennel bulb and remove the green parts. Wash the bulb and cut into small pieces. Set aside.

Rinse the collard greens under cold running water. Drain and chop into small pieces. Set aside.

Wash the cucumber and cut into thin slices. Fill the measuring cup and reserve the rest for later. Set aside.

Peel the lemon and cut lengthwise in half. Set aside.

Now, combine fennel, collard greens, cucumber, and lemon in a juicer and process until juiced. Transfer to a serving glass and stir in the water and cayenne pepper.

Refrigerate for 20 minutes before serving.

Enjoy!

Nutritional information per serving: Kcal: 68, Protein: 4.9g, Carbs: 26.3g, Fats: 0.9g

18. Mango Peach Juice

Ingredients:

1 cup of mango, chunked

1 medium-sized peach, chopped

1 large banana, chunked

1 large orange, peeled

¼ tsp of cinnamon, ground

Preparation:

Peel the mango and cut into small chunks. Fill the measuring cup and reserve the rest for later. Set aside.

Wash the peach and cut lengthwise in half. Remove the pit and cut into small pieces. Set aside.

Peel the banana and cut into small chunks. Set aside.

Peel the orange and divide into wedges. Cut each wedge in half and set aside.

Now, combine mango, peach, banana, and orange in a juicer. Process until well juiced. Transfer to a serving glass and stir in the cinnamon.

Add some crushed ice and serve immediately.

Enjoy!

Nutritional information per serving: Kcal: 313, Protein: 5.9g, Carbs: 91.7g, Fats: 1.6g

19. Tomato Spinach Juice

Ingredients:

1 medium-sized tomato, chopped

1 cup of fresh spinach, torn

1 whole lemon, peeled

1 large red bell pepper, chopped

1 tsp of rosemary, finely chopped

Preparation:

Wash the tomato and place in a small bowl. Chop into small pieces and reserve the tomato juice while cutting. Set aside.

Wash the spinach thoroughly under cold running water. Drain and torn into small pieces. Set aside.

Peel the lemon and cut lengthwise in half. Set aside.

Wash the bell pepper and cut in half. Remove the stem and seeds. Cut into small pieces and set aside.

Now, combine tomato, spinach, lemon, and bell pepper in a juicer and process until juiced. Transfer to a serving glass and stir in the rosemary.

Add few ice cubes and serve immediately.

Nutritional information per serving: Kcal: 92, Protein: 9.3g, Carbs: 27.7g, Fats: 1.7g

20. Avocado Lettuce Juice

Ingredients:

1 cup of avocado, chunked

1 cup of red leaf lettuce, shredded

1 large banana, sliced

½ cup of strawberries, chopped

1 small Red Delicious apple, cored

¼ tsp of cinnamon, ground

Preparation:

Peel the avocado and cut lengthwise in half. Remove the pit and chop into small pieces. Set aside.

Wash the lettuce thoroughly under cold running water. Drain and chop into small pieces. Set aside.

Peel the banana and chop into small pieces. Set aside.

Wash the strawberries and remove the stems. Cut into bite-sized pieces and fill the measuring cup. Set aside.

Now, combine avocado, lettuce, banana, and strawberries in a juicer and process until juiced. Transfer to a serving glass and stir in the cinnamon.

Add some ice and serve immediately.

Enjoy!

Nutritional information per serving: Kcal: 405, Protein: 5.7g, Carbs: 72.2g, Fats: 23.1g

21. Apricot Strawberry Juice

Ingredients:

1 cup of apricots, chopped

1 cup of strawberries, chopped

1 cup of celery, chopped

1 small Golden Delicious apple, cored

¼ tsp of cinnamon, ground

Preparation:

Wash the apricots and cut in half. Remove the pits and chop into small pieces. Fill the measuring cup and reserve the rest for later. Set aside.

Wash the strawberries and remove the stems. Cut into small pieces and fill the measuring cup. Reserve the rest for later.

Wash the celery and chop into small pieces. Set aside.

Wash the apple and cut lengthwise in half. Remove the core and cut into small pieces. Set aside.

Now, combine apricots, strawberries, celery, and apple in a juicer and process until juiced. Transfer to a serving glass and stir in the cinnamon.

Add some ice and serve immediately.

Nutritional information per serving: Kcal: 170, Protein: 4.3g, Carbs: 49.9g, Fats: 1.4g

22. Mint Melon Juice

Ingredients:

1 cup of watermelon, chopped

1 large banana, chopped

1 whole lime, peeled

1 cup of fresh mint, torn

1 small Granny Smith's apple, cored

¼ tsp of cinnamon, ground

Preparation:

Cut the watermelon in half. Cut one large wedge and wrap the rest in a plastic foil and refrigerate. Peel the slice and cut into small cubes. Remove the pits and fill the measuring cup. Set aside.

Peel the banana and cut into small chunks. Set aside.

Peel the lime and cut lengthwise in half. Set aside.

Wash the mint thoroughly under cold running water. Drain and torn into small pieces. Set aside.

Wash the apple and cut lengthwise in half. Remove the core and chop into bite-sized pieces. Set aside.

Now, combine watermelon, banana, lime, mint, and apple in a juicer and process until juiced. Transfer to a serving glass and stir in the cinnamon.

Add some crushed ice and serve immediately.

Nutritional information per serving: Kcal: 239, Protein: 4.2g, Carbs: 69.5g, Fats: 1.2g

23. Brussels Sprout Artichoke Juice

Ingredients:

2 cups of Brussels sprouts, halved

1 large artichoke, chopped

1 cup of cucumber, sliced

¼ tsp of turmeric, ground

¼ tsp of ginger, ground

2 oz of water

Preparation:

Wash the Brussels sprouts and trim off the outer layers. Cut each sprout in half and fill the measuring cups. Set aside.

Trim off the outer leaves of the artichoke. Cut into small pieces and set aside.

Wash the cucumber and cut into thin slices. Fill the measuring cup and reserve the rest in the refrigerator.

Now, combine Brussels sprouts, artichoke, and cucumber in a juicer and process until well juiced. Transfer to a serving glass and stir in the ginger, turmeric, and water.

Refrigerate for 15 minutes before serving.

Enjoy!

Nutritional information per serving: Kcal: 98, Protein: 11.6g, Carbs: 34.7g, Fats: 0.8g

24. Strawberry Pear Juice

Ingredients:

1 cup of strawberries, chopped

1 large pear, chopped

1 cup of blackberries

1 small Red Delicious apple, cored

¼ tsp of cinnamon, ground

1 oz of water

Preparation:

Wash the strawberries and remove the stems. Cut into small pieces and fill the measuring cup. Reserve the rest in the refrigerator.

Wash the pear and cut in half. Remove the core and cut into small pieces. Set aside.

Wash the blackberries using a colander. Drain and set aside.

Wash the apple and cut lengthwise in half. Remove the core and chop into bite-sized pieces. Set aside.

Now, combine strawberries, pear, blackberries, and apple in a juicer and process until well juiced. Transfer to a serving glass and stir in the cinnamon.

Refrigerate for 15 minutes before serving.

Enjoy!

Nutritional information per serving: Kcal: 246, Protein: 4.2g, Carbs: 82.1g, Fats: 1.7g

25. Spinach Honeydew Melon Juice

Ingredients:

1 cup of spinach, chopped

1 medium-sized wedge of honeydew melon

1 cup of raspberries

1 small Golden Delicious apple, cored

¼ tsp of ginger, ground

Preparation:

Wash the spinach thoroughly under cold running water. Drain and chop into small pieces. Set aside.

Cut melon lengthwise in half. Scoop out the seeds and then wash the melon. Cut one wedge and peel it. Cut into bite-sized pieces and set aside. Reserve the rest in the refrigerator.

Place the raspberries in a colander and rinse well under cold running water. Drain and set aside.

Wash the apple and cut lengthwise in half. Remove the core and cut into bite-sized pieces. Set aside.

Now, combine spinach, melon, raspberries, and apple in a juicer and process until juiced. Transfer to a serving glass and stir in the ginger. Add some ice before serving.

Enjoy!

Nutritional information per serving: Kcal: 142, Protein: 4.5g, Carbs: 46.1g, Fats: 1.4g

26. Orange Fennel Juice

Ingredients:

1 large orange, peeled

1 cup of fennel, chopped

1 small Granny Smith's apple, cored

1 cup of blueberries

¼ tsp of ginger, ground

Preparation:

Peel the orange and divide into wedges. Cut each wedge in half and set aside.

Trim off the outer wilted layers of the fennel. Roughly chop it and fill the measuring cup. Reserve the rest for later.

Wash the apple and cut lengthwise in half. Remove the core and cut into bite-sized pieces. Set aside.

Place the blueberries in a colander and wash thoroughly under cold running water. Drain and set aside.

Now, combine orange, fennel, apple, and blueberries in a juicer and process until juiced. Transfer to a serving glass and stir in the ginger.

Add few ice cubes and serve immediately.

Enjoy!

Nutritional information per serving: Kcal: 222, Protein: 4.5g, Carbs: 69.1g, Fats: 1.5g

27. Raspberry Blueberry Juice

Ingredients:

2 cups of raspberries

1 cup of blueberries

1 medium-sized zucchini, sliced

1 small ginger knob, peeled

1 oz of coconut water

Preparation:

Combine raspberries and blueberries in a large colander. Rinse well under cold running water. Drain and set aside.

Wash the zucchini and cut into thin slices. Set aside.

Peel the ginger knob and cut into small pieces. Set aside.

Now, combine raspberries, blueberries, zucchini, and ginger in a juicer and process until juiced. Transfer to a serving glass and stir in the coconut water.

Add crushed ice or refrigerate for 15 minutes before serving.

Enjoy!

Nutritional information per serving: Kcal: 164, Protein: 6.5g, Carbs: 58g, Fats: 2.7g

28. Sweet Potato Lemon Juice

Ingredients:

1 cup of sweet potato, cubed

1 whole lemon, peeled

1 cup of fresh spinach, torn

1 cup of pomegranate seeds

2 oz of water

Preparation:

Peel the sweet potato and cut into small cubes. Place in a deep pot and add 3 cups of water. Bring it to a boil and cook for 5 minutes. Remove from the heat and drain. Set aside.

Peel the lemon and cut lengthwise in half. Set aside.

Wash the spinach thoroughly under cold running water. Drain and torn into small pieces. Set aside.

Cut the top of the pomegranate fruit using a sharp paring knife. Slice down to each of the white membranes inside of the fruit. Pop the seeds into a measuring cup and set aside.

Now, combine previously cooked potato, lemon, spinach, and pomegranate seeds in a juicer. Process until well juiced.

Transfer to a serving glass and stir in the water. Add some ice and serve immediately.

Enjoy!

Nutritional information per serving: Kcal: 195, Protein: 10.2g, Carbs: 56.1g, Fats: 2.1g

29. Broccoli Kale Juice

Ingredients:

2 cups of broccoli, chopped

2 cups of kale, chopped

1 cup of cucumber, sliced

1 whole lime, peeled and halved

1 whole lemon, peeled and halved

1 oz of water

Preparation:

Wash the broccoli and trim off the outer leaves. Cut into small pieces and fill the measuring cup. Reserve the rest in the refrigerator.

Wash the kale thoroughly under cold running water. Drain and chop into small pieces. Set aside.

Wash the cucumber and cut into thin slices. Fill the measuring cup and reserve the rest for later.

Peel the lime and lemon. Cut each fruit lengthwise in half and set aside.

Now, combine broccoli, kale, cucumber, lime, and lemon in a juicer and process until juiced. Transfer to a serving glass and stir in the water.

Sprinkle with some mint for some extra taste, but it's optional.

Refrigerate for 10 minutes before serving.

Enjoy!

Nutritional information per serving: Kcal: 116, Protein: 12.1g, Carbs: 34.8g, Fats: 2.2g

30. Mango Peach Juice

Ingredients:

1 cup of mango, chopped

1 large peach, chopped

1 whole plum, chopped

1 small Red Delicious apple, cored

1 oz of coconut water

Preparation:

Peel the mango and cut into small cubes. Fill the measuring cup and reserve the rest for later.

Wash the peach and cut lengthwise in half. Remove the pit and cut into small pieces. Set aside.

Wash the plum and cut in half. Remove the pit and chop into small pieces. Set aside.

Wash the apple cut lengthwise in half. Remove the core and chop into small pieces. Set aside.

Now, combine mango, peach, plum, and apple in a juicer and process until juiced. Transfer to a serving glass and stir in the coconut water.

Add some ice and serve immediately.

Nutritional information per serving: Kcal: 252, Protein: 3.8g, Carbs: 71.1g, Fats: 1.6g

31. Strawberry Watermelon Juice

Ingredients:

1 cup of strawberries, chopped

1 large wedge of watermelon

1 large banana, sliced

2 whole plums, pitted

Preparation:

Wash the strawberries and remove the stems. Cut into small pieces and fill the measuring cup. Reserve the rest for in the refrigerator.

Cut the watermelon in half. Cut one large wedge and wrap the rest in a plastic foil and refrigerate. Peel the slice and cut into small cubes. Remove the pits and fill the measuring cup. Set aside.

Peel the banana and cut into thin slices. Set aside.

Wash the plums and cut into halves. Remove the pits and cut into small pieces. Set aside.

Now, combine strawberries, watermelon, banana, and plums in a juicer and process until juiced. Transfer to a serving glass and add some ice.

Serve immediately.

Nutritional information per serving: Kcal: 273, Protein: 5.1g, Carbs: 78.8g, Fats: 1.6g

32. Cantaloupe Blackberry Juice

Ingredients:

1 cup of cantaloupe, chopped

1 cup of blackberries

2 whole kiwis, peeled

1 small green apple, cored

¼ tsp of ginger, ground

Preparation:

Cut the cantaloupe in half. Scrape out the seeds and cut one one large wedge. Peel and chop into small pieces. Wrap the rest in a plastic foil and refrigerate for later.

Place the blackberries in a colander. Rinse well under cold running water and drain. Set aside.

Peel the kiwi and cut in half. Set aside.

Wash the apple and cut lengthwise in half. Remove the core and cut into bite-sized pieces. Set aside.

Now, combine cantaloupe, blackberries, kiwi, and apple in a juicer and process until juiced. Transfer to a serving glass and stir in the ginger.

Add few ice cubes and serve immediately.

Nutritional information per serving: Kcal: 181, Protein: 4.7g, Carbs: 56.3g, Fats: 1.6g

33. Lemon Pineapple Juice

Ingredients:

1 whole lemon, peeled

1 cup of pineapple, chunked

1 whole grapefruit, peeled and wedged

1 cup of black grapes

¼ tsp of cinnamon, ground

Preparation:

Peel the lemon and cut lengthwise in half. Set aside.

Using a sharp paring knife, cut the top of the pineapple. Gently remove all hard skin and cut into chunks. Fill the measuring cup and reserve the in the refrigerator.

Peel the grapefruit and divide into wedges. Cut each wedge in half and set aside.

Rinse the grapes thoroughly under cold running water. Remove the stems and fill the measuring cup. Set aside.

Now, combine lemon, pineapple, grapefruit, and grapes in a juicer and process until juiced. Transfer to a serving glass and stir in the cinnamon.

Add some crushed ice and serve immediately.

Nutritional information per serving: Kcal: 230, Protein: 4g, Carbs: 69.1g, Fats: 1.1g

34. Pomegranate Blueberry Juice

Ingredients:

1 cup of pomegranate seeds

1 cup of blueberries

1 whole lime, peeled

1 small Granny Smith's apple, cored

¼ tsp of ginger, ground

2 oz of water

Preparation:

Cut the top of the pomegranate fruit using a sharp paring knife. Slice down to each of the white membranes inside of the fruit. Pop the seeds into a measuring cup and set aside.

Place the blueberries in a colander. Rinse well under cold running water and drain. Set aside.

Peel the lime and cut lengthwise in half. Set aside.

Wash the apple and cut lengthwise in half. Remove the core and cut into bite-sized pieces and set aside.

Now, combine pomegranate seeds, blueberries, lime, and apple in a juicer and process until juiced. Transfer to a serving glass and stir in the ginger and water.

Refrigerate for 10 minutes before serving.

Enjoy!

Nutritional information per serving: Kcal: 206, Protein: 3.3g, Carbs: 61.1g, Fats: 1.8g

35. Peach Beet Juice

Ingredients:

1 large peach, pitted and chopped

1 cup of beets, trimmed and sliced

1 cup of apricots, sliced

1 whole lemon, peeled and halved

1 small ginger slice, peeled

1 oz of water

Preparation:

Wash the peach and cut lengthwise in half. Remove the pit and chop into bite-sized pieces. Set aside.

Wash the beets and trim off the green ends. Slightly peel and cut into thin slices. Fill the measuring cup and reserve the rest for later.

Wash the apricots and cut lengthwise in half. Remove the pits and cut into thin slices. Fill the measuring cup and reserve the rest in the refrigerator.

Peel the ginger slice and chop into small pieces. Set aside.

Now, combine peach, beets, apricots, lemon, and ginger in a juicer and process until juiced. Transfer to a serving glass and stir in the water.

Refrigerate for 15 minutes before serving.

Nutritional information per serving: Kcal: 180, Protein: 6.7g, Carbs: 53.8g, Fats: 1.5g

36. Apple Cherry Juice

Ingredients:

1 small Golden Delicious apple, cored

1 cup of cherries

1 cup of celery, chopped

1 whole plum, pitted and chopped

¼ tsp of cinnamon, ground

2 tbsp of coconut water

Preparation:

Wash the apple and cut lengthwise in half. Remove the core and cut into bite-sized pieces. Set aside.

Wash the cherries using a colander. Drain and cut each in half. Remove the pits and set aside.

Now, combine apple, cherries, celery, and plum in a juicer and process until juiced. Transfer to a serving glass and stir in the cinnamon and coconut water.

Add some crushed ice and serve immediately.

Nutritional information per serving: Kcal: 182, Protein: 3.1g, Carbs: 52.7g, Fats: 0.8g

37. Fennel Bell Pepper Juice

Ingredients:

1 cup of fennel, sliced

1 large yellow bell pepper, chopped

1 cup of Romaine lettuce, chopped

1 cup of cucumber, sliced

1 small zucchini, cubed

Preparation:

Trim off the fennel bulb and remove the green parts. Wash it and cut into small pieces. Fill the measuring cup and reserve the rest for later. Set aside.

Wash the bell pepper and cut lengthwise in half. Remove the stem and seeds. Cut into small pieces and set aside.

Wash the Romaine lettuce thoroughly under cold running water. Drain and chop into small pieces. Set aside.

Wash the cucumber and cut into thin slices. Fill the measuring cup and reserve the rest for later.

Wash the zucchini and cut into small cubes. Set aside.

Now, combine fennel, bell pepper, lettuce, cucumber, and zucchini in a juicer and process until juiced. Transfer to a serving glass and refrigerate for 10 minutes before serving.

Nutritional information per serving: Kcal: 85, Protein: 5.3g, Carbs: 25.2g, Fats: 1.1g

38. Tomato Asparagus Juice

Ingredients:

1 medium-sized tomato, chopped

1 cup of asparagus, trimmed and chopped

1 cup of collard greens, torn

1 cup of spinach, torn

¼ tsp salt

1 rosemary sprig

Preparation:

Wash the tomato and place it in a small bowl. Cut into small pieces and reserve the tomato juice while cutting. Set aside.

Wash the asparagus and trim off the woody ends. Cut into small pieces and fill the measuring cup. Set aside.

Combine collard greens and spinach in a large colander. Wash under cold running water and drain. Torn into small pieces and set aside.

Now, combine tomato, asparagus, collard greens, and spinach in a juicer and process until juiced. Transfer to a serving glass and stir in the reserve tomato juice and salt. Sprinkle with rosemary.

You can add some basil for some extra taste, but it's optional.

Serve immediately.

Nutritional information per serving: Kcal: 66, Protein: 11.2g, Carbs: 19.6g, Fats: 1.5g

39.   Orange Broccoli Juice

Ingredients:

1 large orange, peeled

1 cup of broccoli, chopped

1 cup of cucumber, sliced

1 whole lime, peeled and halved

2 oz of coconut water

¼ tsp of ginger, ground

Preparation:

Peel the orange and divide into wedges. Cut each wedge in half and set aside.

Wash the broccoli and trim off the outer leaves. Cut into small pieces and fill the measuring cup. Reserve the rest in the refrigerator.

Wash the cucumber and cut into thin slices. Fill the measuring cup and reserve the rest for later.

Peel the lime and cut lengthwise in half. Set aside.

Now, combine orange, broccoli, cucumber, and lime in a juicer and process until juiced. Transfer to a serving glass and stir in the coconut water and ginger. Add some ice and serve immediately.

Nutritional information per serving: Kcal: 106, Protein: 4.8g, Carbs: 33.3g, Fats: 0.6g

40. Guava Strawberry Juice

Ingredients:

1 whole guava, chunked

1 cup of strawberries, chopped

1 small Granny Smith's apple, cored and chopped

1 whole lemon, peeled and halved

¼ tsp of ginger, ground

2 oz of water

Preparation:

Peel the guava and cut in half. Scoop out the seeds and wash it. Cut into small chunks and set aside.

Wash the strawberries and remove the stems. Cut into small pieces and fill the measuring cup. Reserve the rest in the refrigerator. Set aside.

Wash the apple and cut lengthwise in half. Remove the core and cut into bite-sized pieces. Set aside.

Peel the lemon and cut lengthwise in half. Set aside.

Now, combine guava, strawberries, apple, and lemon in a juicer and process until juiced. Transfer to a serving glass and stir in the ginger and water.

Refrigerate for 15 minutes before serving.

Enjoy!

Nutritional information per serving: Kcal: 136, Protein: 3.6g, Carbs: 43.9g, Fats: 1.3g

41. Banana Mint Juice

Ingredients:

2 large bananas, peeled and chopped

1 cup of fresh mint, torn

1 whole kiwi, peeled

1 whole lemon, peeled

1 large Red Delicious apple, cored and chopped

¼ tsp of cinnamon, ground

Preparation:

Peel the bananas and cut into small pieces. Set aside.

Wash the mint thoroughly under cold running water. Drain and torn into small pieces. Set aside.

Wash the apple and cut lengthwise in half. Remove the core and cut into bite-sized pieces. Set aside.

Now, combine bananas, mint, kiwi, lemon, and apple in a juicer and process until well juiced. Transfer to a serving glass and stir in the cinnamon.

Add some ice and serve immediately.

Enjoy!

Nutritional information per serving: Kcal: 398, Protein: 6.1g, Carbs: 117g, Fats: 2.1g

42. Carrot Celery Juice

Ingredients:

2 large carrots, chunked

1 cup of celery, chopped

1 whole grapefruit, peeled

1 small Golden Delicious apple, cored and chopped

¼ tsp of cinnamon, ground

Preparation:

Wash and peel the carrots. Cut into small chunks and set aside.

Wash the celery and cut into small pieces. Fill the measuring cup and reserve the rest in the refrigerator.

Peel the grapefruit and divide into wedges. Cut each wedge in half and set aside.

Wash the apple and cut lengthwise in half. Remove the core and cut into bite-sized pieces. Set aside.

Now, combine carrots, celery, grapefruit, and apple in a juicer and process until well juiced. Transfer to a serving glass and stir in the cinnamon.

Add some crushed ice and serve immediately.

Enjoy!

Nutritional information per serving: Kcal: 203, Protein: 4.3g, Carbs: 60.6g, Fats: 1.1g

43. Leek Pear Juice

Ingredients:

1 whole leek, chopped

1 medium-sized pear, chopped

1 whole lime, peeled

1 cup of cantaloupe, peeled and chopped

1 oz of coconut water

¼ tsp of ginger, ground

Preparation:

Wash the leek thoroughly under cold running water. Drain and chop into small pieces. Set aside.

Wash the pear lengthwise in half. Remove the core and cut into bite-sized pieces. Set aside.

Peel the lime and cut lengthwise in half. Set aside.

Cut the cantaloupe in half. Scoop out the seeds and flesh. Cut and peel one large wedge. Chop into chunks and fill the measuring cup. Reserve the rest of the cantaloupe in a refrigerator.

Now, combine leek, pear, lime, and cantaloupe in a juicer and process until juiced. Transfer to a serving glass and stir in the coconut water and ginger.

Add some ice, or refrigerate for 10 minutes before serving.

Nutritional information per serving: Kcal: 184, Protein: 3.5g, Carbs: 56.2g, Fats: 0.8g

44. Artichoke Basil Juice

Ingredients:

1 medium-sized artichoke, chopped

1 cup of fresh basil, torn

1 cup of red leaf lettuce, chopped

1 cup of purple cabbage, chopped

1 cup of cucumber, sliced

1 large carrot, sliced

Preparation:

Trim off the outer layers of the artichoke using a sharp paring knife. Cut into bite-sized pieces and set aside.

Rinse the basil with cold water and torn into small pieces. Set aside.

Combine lettuce and cabbage in a large colander and rinse well under cold running water. Drain and chop into small pieces. Set aside.

Wash the cucumber and cut into thin slices. Fill the measuring cup and reserve the rest in the refrigerator.

Wash and peel the carrot. Cut into thin slices and set aside.

Now, combine artichoke, basil, lettuce, cabbage, cucumber, and carrot in a juicer and process until juiced. Transfer to a serving glass and serve immediately.

Nutritional information per serving: Kcal: 88, Protein: 7.6g, Carbs: 30.1g, Fats: 0.7g

45. Avocado Plum Juice

Ingredients:

1 cup of avocado, cubed

2 whole plums, chopped

1 whole lime, pitted and chopped

1 small pear, chopped

2 oz of coconut water

¼ tsp of ginger, ground

Preparation:

Peel the avocado and cut lengthwise in half. Remove the pit and cut into small cubes. Fill the measuring cup and reserve the rest for later.

Wash the plums and cut in half. Remove the pits and cut into small pieces. Set aside.

Peel the lime and cut lengthwise in half. Set aside.

Wash the pear and cut in half. Remove the core and into bite-sized pieces. Set side.

Now, combine avocado, plums, lime, and pear in a juicer and process until juiced. Transfer to a serving glass and stir in the coconut water and ginger.

Add some ice and serve immediately.

Nutritional information per serving: Kcal: 328, Protein: 4.6g, Carbs: 54.1g, Fats: 22.6g

46. Brussels Sprout Carrot Juice

Ingredients:

2 cups of Brussels sprouts, halved

2 large radishes, chopped

1 small zucchini, chopped

1 cup of cucumber, sliced

2 large carrots, sliced

¼ tsp of turmeric, ground

Preparation:

Wash the Brussels sprouts and trim off the outer layers. Cut into halves and fill the measuring cups. Reserve the rest in the refrigerator.

Wash the radishes and trim off the green parts. Slightly peel and cut into small pieces. Set aside.

Wash the zucchini and cut into thin slices. Set aside.

Wash the cucumber and cut into thin slices. Fill the measuring cup and reserve the rest for later.

Wash and peel the carrots. Cut into thin slices and set aside.

Now, combine Brussels sprouts, radishes, zucchini, cucumber, and carrots in a juicer and process until juiced. Transfer to a serving glass and stir in the turmeric. Refrigerate for 15 minutes before serving.

Nutritional information per serving: Kcal: 118, Protein: 9.2g, Carbs: 35.7g, Fats: 1.3g

MEALS

1. Portobello Spinach Mushrooms

Ingredients:

4 large Portobello mushrooms, stems removed

4 tbsp. of balsamic vinegar

1 tbsp. of olive oil

1 tsp of dried basil, minced

1 garlic clove, crushed

1 tsp of dried oregano, ground

1 cup of fresh spinach, chopped

1 tbsp. of butter

½ tsp of salt

3 tbsp. of Parmesan cheese, shredded

Preparation:

Preheat the oil in a large frying pan over a medium-high temperature. Add garlic and stir-fry for 2 minutes, or until translucent. Add mushrooms and cook for 5 minutes, or until nicely browned. Remove from the heat and set aside.

Meanwhile, combine vinegar, basil, and oregano in a mixing bowl. Whisk well to blend and set aside.

Melt the butter in a frying pan and add spinach. Sprinkle with some salt and cook for 3-4 minutes or until nicely tender. Remove from the heat and set aside.

Stuff the mushrooms with spinach and transfer to serving plate. Drizzle with previously made dressing and sprinkle Parmesan cheese.

Serve immediately.

Nutritional information per serving: Kcal: 207, Protein: 9.4g, Carbs: 4.1g, Fats: 17.9g

2.   Zucchini Omelet

Ingredients:

6 large eggs, beaten

2 cups of zucchini, shredded

1 tbsp. of olive oil

½ cup of button mushrooms, chopped

½ tsp of Himalayan salt

¼ tsp of black pepper, ground

Preparation:

Preheat the oil in a large skillet over a medium-high temperature. Add zucchini and mushrooms. Cook for 5 minutes, or until nicely tender.

Meanwhile, whisk the eggs, salt, and pepper in a mixing bowl. Pour this mixture over the vegetables. Stir until eggs coat all well. Cook for about 3-4 minutes or until eggs are set. Remove from the heat.

Sprinkle with fresh parsley and serve.

Nutritional information per serving: Kcal: 198, Protein: 13.9g, Carbs: 3.8g, Fats: 14.8g

3. Garbanzo Casserole

Ingredients:

2 cups of chicken broth, unsalted

1 medium-sized carrot, sliced

½ cup of barley, soaked overnight

2 cups of garbanzo beans, pre-cooked

1 small red onion, chopped

4 tbsp. of fresh parsley, finely chopped

1 garlic clove, crushed

½ tsp of salt

Preparation:

Preheat the oven to 375°F.

Soak the beans overnight.

Drain and rinse the beans. Place them in a pot of boiling water and cook until soften. Remove from the heat and drain. Set aside.

Now, combine beans, carrot, barley, onion, garlic, and salt in a large bowl. Stir all well to combine and transfer to casserole dish. Pour over the broth and sprinkle with parsley.

Cover with a lid or wrap with aluminum foil. Place it in the oven and bake for about 40-45 minutes.

Remove from the oven and let it cool for a while before serving.

Nutritional information per serving: Kcal: 198, Protein: 13.9g, Carbs: 3.8g, Fats: 14.8g

4. Green Tea Porridge

Ingredients:

1 cup of white quinoa

1 cup of water

1 tsp of matcha green tea powder

1 tbsp. of maple syrup,

¼ cup of dates, chopped

1 cup of coconut milk

1 tsp of vanilla extract

Preparation:

Combine water and quinoa in a deep pot. Bring it to a boil, then reduce the heat to low and add dates and matcha green tea powder. Cover with a lid and cook for about 15-20 minutes.

Now, pour the coconut milk and stir in the vanilla extract and maple syrup. Cook for 3 minutes and remove from the heat.

Nutritional information per serving: Kcal: 456, Protein: 10.2g, Carbs: 56.6g, Fats: 22.6g

5. Basmati & Beans

Ingredients:

1 cup of basmati rice, pre-cooked

3 cups of water

1 medium-sized celery stalk, chopped

¼ cup of spring onions, chopped

1 medium-sized bell pepper, chopped

1 lb. of kidney beans, pre-cooked

2 cups of tomatoes, diced

2 garlic cloves, crushed

¼ tsp of Tabasco sauce

1 tbsp. of olive oil

¼ tsp of black pepper, ground

Preparation:

Place the rice in a deep pot. Add 3 cups of water and bring it to a boil. Reduce the heat to low and cook for 15 minutes more, or until liquid is absorbed. Remove from the heat and set aside.

Preheat the oil in a large skillet over a medium-high temperature. Add celery, spring onions, and bell pepper. Cook for about 3-4 minutes then reduce the heat to low. Cook for another 3 minutes then add tomatoes, beans and sprinkle with salt and pepper.

Bring it to a boil and reduce the heat to low. Cover with a lid and cook for 10 more minutes. Stir in the rice and cook for 2 minutes. Remove from the heat and serve.

Nutritional information per serving: Kcal: 272, Protein: 13.4g, Carbs: 50.4g, Fats: 2.4g

6. Strawberry Kale Smoothie

Ingredients:

1 cup of fresh kale, organic

½ cup of frozen strawberries, chopped

½ cup of plums, pitted and chopped

1 cup of coconut water

1 tbsp. of hemp oil

1 tbsp. of chia seeds

Preparation:

Wash the kale thoroughly under cold running water. Roughly chop it and set aside.

Wash the plums and remove the pit. Chop it and set aside.

Now, combine kale, plums, and strawberries in a food processor. Add coconut water, hemp oil and blend until nicely smooth. Transfer to serving glasses and sprinkle with chia seeds.

Refrigerate for 20 minutes, or add some ice cubes and serve immediately.

Nutritional information per serving: Kcal: 194, Protein: 1.9g, Carbs: 10.2g, Fats: 15.3g

7. Orzo Cod Stew

Ingredients:

12 oz. of cod fillets, boneless and chopped

2 cups of chicken broth

2 cups of canned tomatoes

4 oz. of orzo pasta, pre-cooked

1 small onion, chopped

¼ tsp of black pepper, ground

¼ tsp of turmeric, ground

½ tsp of garlic powder

2 tsp of olive oil

½ tsp of salt

Preparation:

Cook pasta using package instructions. Remove from the heat and drain well. Set aside.

Preheat the oil in a large nonstick frying pan over a medium-high temperature. Add onion and garlic powder and stir-fry until translucent.

Now, add tomatoes and vegetable broth. Sprinkle with salt, pepper, and turmeric. Stir well and reduce the heat to low. Cook for about 7-10 minutes then add chopped fish.

Cook for 5-10 minutes, or until fish is cooked. Remove from the heat and stir in the pasta.

Serve warm.

Nutritional information per serving: Kcal: 135, Protein: 14.9g, Carbs: 12.3g, Fats: 2.6g

8.   Creamy Fuji Peach Salad

Ingredients:

1 large peach, pitted and chopped

2 apricots, pitted and chopped

1 large banana, chopped

1 cup of watermelon

1 large Fuji apple, cored and chopped

4 tbsp. of coconut water

1 tsp of agave nectar

2 tbsp. of sour cream

2 tbsp. of lemon juice

1 tbsp. of lemon zest

Preparation:

Mix together sour cream, lemon juice, coconut water, and agave nectar in a mixing bowl. Stir well to blend and set aside to allow flavors to meld.

Combine peach apricots, banana, watermelon, and apple in a large salad bowl. Drizzle with previously made dressing and stir well to coat.

Refrigerate for 30 minutes before serving.

Enjoy!

Nutritional information per serving: Kcal: 146, Protein: 2.1g, Carbs: 32.6g, Fats: 2.4g

9. Oven-Baked Crispy Chicken

Ingredients:

1 lb. of chicken breasts, skinless and boneless

¼ cup of tomatoes, sun-dried

½ cup of breadcrumbs

1 tsp of Italian seasoning

2 garlic cloves, minced

1 free-range egg, beaten

¼ tsp of black pepper, ground

½ tsp of salt

1 tbsp. of fresh rosemary, finely chopped

2 tbsp. of olive oil

Preparation:

Preheat the oven to 400°F.

Combine tomatoes, breadcrumbs, Italian seasoning, and garlic in a food processor and process until nicely blended. Transfer this mixture to a large bowl.

Now, dip the chicken breasts in egg, then in breadcrumbs mixture.

Take a large baking sheet and grease it with oil. Spread the chicken breasts in it and place it in the oven.

Bake for about 20-25 minutes or until golden brown. Remove from the oven and sprinkle with fresh rosemary.

Serve immediately.

Nutritional information per serving: Kcal: 474, Protein: 48.3g, Carbs: 15.3g, Fats: 23.6g

10. Wild Asparagus Soup

Ingredients:

2 lbs. of wild asparagus, trimmed

2 small onions, peeled and finely chopped

1 cup of heavy cream

4 cups of vegetable broth

2 tbsp of butter

1 tbsp. of vegetable oil

½ tsp of salt

½ tsp of dried oregano, ground

½ tsp of cayenne pepper, ground

Preparation:

Rinse and drain asparagus. Cut into about one inch thick pieces. Set aside.

Melt the butter in a heavy-bottomed pot over a medium-high temperature. Add onions and stir-fry until translucent. Now, add asparagus, oregano, salt, and Cayenne pepper. Stir well and continue to cook until asparagus soften.

Add the vegetable broth and mix well to combine. Bring it to a boil and then reduce the heat to low.

Cover with a lid and cook for 20 minutes. Remove from the heat and stir in the heavy cream.

Serve immediately.

Nutritional information per serving: Kcal: 284, Protein: 11g, Carbs: 14.1g, Fats: 22g

11. Marinara Potato Balls

Ingredients:

3 large potatoes, peeled

1 large onion, peeled and finely chopped

1 lb. fresh spinach, torn

¼ cup of mozzarella cheese, shredded

2 eggs, beaten

½ tsp of salt

¼ tsp of black pepper, freshly ground

1 tsp of dried oregano, minced

1 cup of skim milk

¼ cup of all-purpose flour

¼ cup of corn flour

<u>For homemade marinara (optional):</u>

1 lb. fresh tomatoes, peeled and roughly chopped

1 large onion, peeled and finely chopped

3 garlic cloves, peeled and crushed

4 tbsp. of extra-virgin olive oil

¼ cup of white wine

1 tsp of sugar

1 tbsp. of dried rosemary, crushed

½ tsp of salt

1 tbsp. of tomato paste

Preparation:

First, you will have to prepare the balls.

Place peeled potatoes in a deep, heavy bottomed-pot and add enough water to cover. Bring it to a boil and reduce the heat. Cook until fork-tender, remove from the heat and drain. Add one cup of milk and puree with a potato masher. Transfer to a large bowl.

Gently whisk in the eggs, one at the time and mix well with a spoon. Add the remaining ingredients and mix them using your hands. This can be a bit messy, but it's definitely the best way to combine the ingredients together.

Shape the balls according to your taste. Set aside.

Heat up the olive oil in a large skillet. Add the onions, garlic, and stir-fry until translucent. Now add peeled tomatoes and reduce the heat to minimum. Cook until tender and almost done, about 10 minutes. Pour in about ¼ cup of white wine, add sugar, rosemary, and salt. Stir in 1 tablespoon of tomato paste and mix well. Cook for 5 more minutes. Remove the marinara from the heat and transfer to the instant pot.

Place the potato balls in a nonstick skillet and cook for 10 minutes on medium temperature. Remove from the heat and pour over the marinara sauce.

Serve immediately.

Nutritional information per serving: Kcal: 434, Protein: 13.3g, Carbs: 61.9g, Fats: 16.1g

12. Baked Root Vegetables

Ingredients:

3 cups of sweet potatoes, peeled and cubed

2 cups of parsnips, peeled and chopped

1 large red onion, chopped

10 oz. of radishes, trimmed and chopped

5 garlic cloves, peeled and crushed

2 tbsp. of olive oil

1 tsp of dried thyme, minced

½ tsp of black pepper, ground

½ tsp of salt

Preparation:

Preheat the oven to 450°F.

Combine potatoes, onion, parsnips, garlic, and radishes in a large bowl. Sprinkle with salt and pepper. Drizzle with olive oil and toss well to coat.

Take a large baking sheet and spread the vegetables in one large layer.

Place it in the oven and bake for about 40-45 minutes. Spoon the vegetables to a serving plate and sprinkle with thyme.

Enjoy!

Nutritional information per serving: Kcal: 184, Protein: 2.5g, Carbs: 33.9g, Fats: 5g

13.   Turkey with Kiwi Pasta

Ingredients:

1 lb. of turkey breasts, cut into bite-sized pieces

8 oz. of noodles, pre-cooked

3 large kiwis, peeled and chopped

2 cups of crookneck squash, chopped

2 cups of broccoli, chopped

4 tbsp. of Parmesan cheese, shredded

2 tbsp. of Dijon mustard

4 tbsp. of red wine vinegar

2 tbsp. of olive oil

1 tbsp. of fresh basil, finely chopped

2 garlic cloves, minced

½ tsp of salt

¼ tsp of black pepper, ground

Preparation:

Preheat 1 tablespoon in a large frying pan over a medium-high temperature. Add meat chops and sprinkle with salt and pepper. Fry for 5 minutes, stirring occasionally. Remove from the heat and set aside.

Cook noodles using package instructions. Stir in the broccoli and crookneck squash in the last minute of noodles cooking. Remove from the heat and drain well. Set aside.

Combine the remaining oil, vinegar, garlic, basil, and mustard in a mixing bowl. Stir well to blend and pour over the noodles mixture. Set aside to cool.

Peel and chop the kiwis and stir in into the noodles.

Serve turkey and spoon over the pasta. Sprinkle with cheese and serve.

Nutritional information per serving: Kcal: 208, Protein: 17g, Carbs: 17.3g, Fats: 8.5g

14. Green Booster Smoothie

Ingredients:

½ cup of broccoli, chopped

½ cup of fresh kale, torn

1 large beet, trimmed and chopped

1 large cucumber, chopped

1 cup of artichoke, chopped

2 oz. of water

½ tsp of Himalayan salt

Preparation:

Wash and prepare the vegetables.

Combine all in a food processor and process until nicely smooth and creamy. Transfer to serving glasses and stir in the water and salt.

Add few ice cubes and serve immediately.

Nutritional information per serving: Kcal: 60, Protein: 3.4g, Carbs: 13.6g, Fats: 0.3g

15. Broccoli Rice Casserole

Ingredients:

10 oz. of fresh broccoli, chopped

1 cup of wild rice, pre-cooked

2 cups of vegetable broth

2 cups of Cheddar cheese, shredded

½ tsp of black pepper, ground

¼ tsp of Cayenne pepper

2 garlic cloves, minced

1 small onion, chopped

1 tbsp. of olive oil

Preparation:

Preheat the oven to 350°F.

Place the rice in a heavy-bottomed pot. Add 3 cups of water and bring it to a boil. Reduce the heat to low and cook for 15 minutes, or until liquid is absorbed. Remove from the heat and set aside.

Spread the broccoli on a large baking sheet in one layer. Steam for 5 minutes and then spread the rice evenly on top.

Meanwhile, combine vegetable broth and cheese in a medium bowl. Sprinkle with pepper and Cayenne pepper. Stir all well to blend and pour over the broccoli and rice.

Place it in the oven and bake for about 35-40 minutes. Remove from the heat and set aside to cool for a while.

Serve warm.

Nutritional information per serving: Kcal: 303, Protein: 16.5g, Carbs: 25.5g, Fats: 15.8g

16. Winter Beef Vegetable Soup

Ingredients:

1 lb. of beef round steak, cut into bite-sized pieces

1 small onion, sliced

2 cups of canned tomatoes

2 medium-sized potatoes, peeled and cubed

1 medium-sized turnip, chopped

1 medium-sized carrot, sliced

½ cup of celery, chopped

½ tsp of black pepper, ground

½ tsp of salt

1 tsp of dried basil, minced

5 cups of water

Preparation:

Place the meat chops and onion in a heavy-bottomed pot. Pour the water and sprinkle with salt, pepper, and basil. Cook until meat is fork-tender.

Now, add tomatoes, potatoes, turnip, and carrot. Reduce the heat to low and cover with a lid. Cook for 20 minutes more and add celery.

Cook for 15 minutes and remove from the heat.

Serve warm.

Nutritional information per serving: Kcal: 303, Protein: 16.5g, Carbs: 25.5g, Fats: 15.8g

17. Quinoa Salmon

Ingredients:

1 lb. of wild salmon fillets, thinly sliced

1 cup of quinoa, pre-cooked

2 garlic cloves, finely chopped

3 cups of water

½ tsp of sea salt

¼ tsp of black pepper, freshly ground

¼ tsp of turmeric, ground

2 tbsp. of olive oil

1 tbsp. of fresh rosemary, finely chopped

2 tbsp. of balsamic vinegar

1 tbsp. of lemon juice, freshly squeezed

Preparation:

Combine quinoa and water in a deep pot. Bring it to a boil, then reduce the heat to low. Cook for another 15 minutes. Remove from the heat and stir in the turmeric. Set aside.

Combine 1 tablespoon of oil, salt, pepper, rosemary, vinegar, and lemon juice in a bowl. Stir well to blend and set aside.

Preheat the remaining oil in a large skillet over a medium-high temperature. Add garlic and stir-fry until translucent. Now, add fillets and cook for 3-4 minutes on each side, or until easily flaked with a fork. Remove from the heat and transfer to serving plate. Drizzle with dressing and serve with quinoa.

Serve immediately.

Nutritional information per serving: Kcal: 256, Protein: 19g, Carbs: 20.6g, Fats: 11.2g

18. Avocado Spinach Salad

Ingredients:

1 cup of avocado chunks

1 cup of spinach, chopped

2 large eggs, hard-boiled

2 tbsp. of lemon juice

1 tbsp. of mayonnaise

½ tsp of Himalayan salt

1 tbsp. of olive oil

¼ tsp of black pepper, ground

Preparation:

Combine lemon juice, mayonnaise, salt, oil, and pepper in a mixing bowl. Stir well and set aside to allow flavors to meld.

Peel the avocado and cut in half. Remove the pit and cut into chunks. set aside.

Hard-boil the eggs. Let it cool and gently peel. Cut into bite-sized pieces and set aside.

Wash the spinach thoroughly and roughly chop it. Set aside.

Now, combine avocado, egg, and spinach in a large salad bowl. Drizzle with dressing and toss well to coat.

Refrigerate for 20 minutes before serving.

Enjoy!

Nutritional information per serving: Kcal: 317, Protein: 8.3g, Carbs: 9.5g, Fats: 8.9g

19. Spinach with Mushrooms

Ingredients:

10 oz. of spinach, chopped

1 cup of button mushrooms, chopped

2 large red bell peppers, sliced

2 garlic cloves, finely chopped

2 tbsp. of olive oil

¼ tsp of chili pepper, ground

½ tsp of Himalayan salt

½ tsp of ginger, ground

Preparation:

Preheat the oil in a large frying pan over a medium-high temperature. add garlic and sprinkle with ginger and chili pepper. Stir-fry for 1 minute.

Now, add mushrooms and sliced bell peppers. Cook for about 3-4 minutes then add spinach. Cook for another 3 minutes and stir constantly. Cook until spinach is wilted.

Serve immediately.

Nutritional information per serving: Kcal: 136, Protein: 4.4g, Carbs: 11.1g, Fats: 10g

20. Breakfast Oatmeal Cake

Ingredients:

2 cups of rolled oats

1 large egg, beaten

3 tbsp. of canola oil

1 tsp of baking powder

¼ cup of prunes

¼ cup of toasted almonds

½ cup of skim milk

2 tbsp. of honey

½ tsp of cinnamon, ground

Preparation:

Preheat the oven to 350°F.

Combine rolled oats, baking powder, almonds, and cinnamon. Stir well and set aside.

Now, whisk egg, canola oil, milk, and honey in a bowl. Whisk well and stir into dry ingredients.

Spread the mixture on large baking sheet in one layer. Place it in the oven and bake for 25 minutes. Spread the prunes and bake for another 5 minutes.

Remove from the oven and serve with milk.

Nutritional information per serving: Kcal: 494, Protein: 12.6g, Carbs: 62.4g, Fats: 23.2g

21. Chicken Pudding with Artichoke

Ingredients:

1 lb. dark and white chicken meat, cooked

2 medium-sized artichokes

2 tbsp. of butter

2 tbsp. of extra-virgin olive oil

1 large lemon, juiced

1 handful of fresh parsley leaves

1 tsp of pink Himalayan salt

¼ tsp of black pepper, freshly ground

½ tsp of chili pepper, ground

Preparation:

Thoroughly rinse the meat and pat dry with a kitchen paper. Using a sharp paring knife, cut the meat into smaller pieces and remove the bones. Rub with olive oil and set aside.

Heat the Sautee pan over medium-high temperature. Turn the heat down slightly to medium and add the meat. Cook for about 1 minute to get it a little golden one side. Then flip each piece, cover with a lid and turn the heat to low. Cook for 10 minutes without removing the lid. Now, turn off the heat and let it sit for another 10 minutes.

Meanwhile, prepare the artichoke. Cut the lemon into halves and squeeze the juice in a small bowl. Divide the juice in half and set aside.

Using a sharp paring knife, trim off the outer leaves until you reach the yellow and soft ones. Cut artichoke into half-inch pieces. Rub with half of the lemon juice and place in a heavy-bottomed pot. Add enough water to cover and cook until completely fork-tender. Remove from the heat and drain. Chill for a while.

Now, combine artichoke with chicken meat in a large bowl. Stir in salt, pepper, and the remaining lemon juice.

Melt the butter over a medium heat and drizzle over pudding. Sprinkle with some chili pepper and parsley. Serve.

Nutritional information per serving: Kcal: 369, Protein: 35.7g, Carbs: 10g, Fats: 21.3g

22. Whole Wheat Chocolate Cookies

Ingredients:

1 cup of whole wheat flour

1 cup of rolled oats

½ cup of pecans, roughly chopped

2 tbsp. of peanut butter

1 cup of chocolate chips, chopped

½ tsp of baking soda

½ cup of honey, raw

3 tbsp. of butter

1 free range egg

Preparation:

Preheat the oven to 375°F.

Combine flour, rolled oats, pecans, and baking soda in a large bowl. Stir well and set aside.

Now, combine peanut butter, chocolate chips, honey, butter and egg. Whisk well all to blend and stir into the dry ingredients. If the butter is not well for shaping, add more flour.

Take a large baking sheet and spoon the cookies in the desired shape. Place it in the oven and bake for 10 minutes. Remove from the oven and let it cool for a while.

Serve with milk or tea.

Nutritional information per serving: Kcal: 287, Protein: 5.3g, Carbs: 40g, Fats: 12.6g

23. Butternut Squash Chili Stew

Ingredients:

1 cup of butternut squash, peeled and chopped

1 cup of black beans, soaked

1 cup of white beans, soaked

1 large red bell pepper, chopped

2 cup of diced tomatoes

2 tbsp. of tomato paste

½ tsp of cumin, ground

¼ tsp of chili pepper, ground

¼ tsp of dried oregano, ground

2 garlic cloves, minced

1 tbsp. of olive oil

½ tsp of salt

Preparation:

Soak the beans overnight.

Drain and place them in a deep pot. Add water to cover and cook until soften. Remove from the heat and drain well. Set aside.

Peel the butternut squash and remove the seeds. Cut into small chunks and place in a deep pot. Add enough water to cover ingredients and cook until tender.

Preheat the oil in a heavy-bottomed pot over a medium-high temperature. Add garlic and stir-fry until translucent. Now, add pepper, beans, tomatoes, and tomato paste. Pour enough water to cover all ingredients and sprinkle with salt.

Bring it to a boil and then reduce the heat. Cover with a lid and cook for about 15-20 minutes. Stir in the squash and cook for 5 minutes more.

Sprinkle with oregano, chili and cumin. Stir well and serve warm.

Nutritional information per serving: Kcal: 332, Protein: 19.4g, Carbs: 58.2g, Fats: 4g

24. Strawberry Pineapple Smoothie

Ingredients:

1 cup of strawberries, chopped

1 cup of pineapple, chopped

¼ cup of coconut milk, organic

½ cup of water

2-3 almonds

1 tsp of honey, raw

Preparation:

Place the strawberries in a colander and wash under cold running water. Drain and remove the green caps and stem. Slice into small pieces and set aside.

Peel the pineapple and cut into chunks.

Now, combine strawberries, pineapple, milk, almonds, honey, and water in a food processor. Process until nicely smooth and add some ice before serving.

Nutritional information per serving: Kcal: 395, Protein: 4.7g, Carbs: 42.4g, Fats: 26.8g

25. Marinated Tuna Steaks

Ingredients:

1 lb. of tuna steaks

4 tbsp. of extra-virgin olive oil

1 tbsp. of balsamic vinegar

1 tsp of lemon juice

1 tbsp. of fresh rosemary, chopped

1 tbsp. of fresh thyme, finely chopped

1 tsp of liquid honey

¼ tsp of cumin, ground

¼ tsp of sea salt

¼ tsp of black pepper, freshly ground

Preparation:

Combine olive oil, vinegar, lemon juice, rosemary, thyme, liquid honey, salt, and pepper in a large bowl. Stir well to blend and place in tuna steaks. Coat well with marinade and set aside for 30 minutes to allow flavors to penetrate into fish.

Preheat the grill over a medium-high heat. Add the tuna steaks and grill for about 2-3 minutes on each side. Brush the marinade while grilling.

Transfer the steak to a serving plate and serve with steamed vegetables.

Nutritional information per serving: Kcal: 454, Protein: 45.4g, Carbs: 3.6g, Fats: 28.5g

26. Broccoli in Lemon Sauce

Ingredients:

1 cup of cauliflower, chopped

2 cups of broccoli, chopped

3 tbsp. of lemon juice, freshly squeezed

1 tbsp. of olive oil

1 garlic clove, crushed

1 tbsp. of fresh parsley, finely chopped

¼ tsp of salt

¼ tsp of black pepper, ground

Preparation:

Wash and cut the broccoli and cauliflower into bite-sized pieces. Spread into one large layer over a large baking sheet. Steam for about 10 minutes over a medium-high temperature. Remove from the oven and transfer to a serving dish. Set aside.

Preheat the oil in a nonstick saucepan over a medium-high temperature. Add garlic and cook for 2 minutes. Now, add lemon juice and cook for another minute. Remove from the heat.

Pour over the lemon juice mixture and stir well to coat. Garnish with some fresh parsley and serve immediately.

Nutritional information per serving: Kcal: 113, Protein: 3.9g, Carbs: 10g, Fats: 7.6g

27. Carrot Raisin Porridge

Ingredients:

1 cup of quinoa

2 cups of water

½ cup of apple juice, unsweetened

1 cup of carrots, grated

3 tbsp. of raisins

1 tbsp. of liquid honey

¼ tsp of cinnamon, ground

½ tsp of vanilla extract

Preparation:

Combine water and quinoa in a medium skillet over a medium high temperature. Bring it to a boil and add apple juice. Reduce the heat to low and cover with a lid. Cook for about 15-20 minutes.

Now, add carrots and raisins. Sprinkle with cinnamon and stir all well. Cook for another 5 minutes and remove from the heat. Stir in the honey and vanilla extract. Top with nuts, but this is optional.

Serve immediately.

Nutritional information per serving: Kcal: 220, Protein: 6.5g, Carbs: 43.4g, Fats: 2.6g

28.   Red Bean Stew

Ingredients:

7 oz. of red beans, pre-cooked

2 medium-sized carrots, chopped

2 celery stalks, chopped

1 large onion, peeled and finely chopped

2 tbsp. of tomato paste

1 tbsp. of all-purpose flour

½ tsp of Cayenne pepper

1 bay leaf

1 cup of vegetable broth

3 tbsp. of extra-virgin olive oil

1 tsp of salt

A handful of fresh parsley

Preparation:

Preheat the oil in a deep pot over a medium-high temperature. Add onion and sauté until translucent. Add celery and carrots and cook for 5 more minutes. Gradually add broth while cooking.

Now, add beans and tomato paste. Sprinkle with Cayenne pepper, salt, and parsley. Stir in the bay leaf.

Stir in the flour and bring it to a boil. Now, reduce the heat to low and cover with a lid. Cook for 40 minutes more and remove from the heat.

Sprinkle with some fresh parsley before serving.

Nutritional information per serving: Kcal: 311, Protein: 13.7g, Carbs: 40.8g, Fats: 11.6g

29. Roma Vegetable Salad

Ingredients:

2 large Roma tomatoes, chopped

1 cup of purple cabbage, shredded

½ cup of fresh spinach, roughly chopped

1 large cucumber, chopped

1 small red bell pepper, chopped

2 garlic cloves, minced

1 small red onion, sliced

3 tbsp. of extra-virgin olive oil

1 tbsp. of red wine vinegar

1 tsp of sea salt

¼ tsp of turmeric, ground

¼ tsp of black pepper, freshly ground

Preparation:

Combine garlic, oil, vinegar, salt, turmeric, and pepper in a mixing bowl. Stir well and set aside for 10 minutes to allow flavors to blend.

Wash the tomatoes and chop into bite-sized pieces. Place them in a large bowl. Set aside.

Combine cabbage and spinach in a colander and wash under cold running water. Shred the cabbage and roughly chop the spinach. Add to the bowl with tomatoes.

Wash the cucumber and pepper and cut into thin slices. You can remove the seeds from pepper, but this is optional.

Peel the onion and chop into thin slices. Add to the bowl with other ingredients.

Now, toss well the vegetables and drizzle with dressing. Toss again to coat all the ingredients.

Serve immediately.

Nutritional information per serving: Kcal: 115, Protein: 1.8g, Carbs: 9.6g, Fats: 8.7g

30. Beef with Potatoes

Ingredients:

1 lb. of sirloin steak, cut into bite-sized pieces

1 tbsp. of olive oil

1 large onion, sliced

½ cup of cherry tomatoes, diced

1 garlic clove

2 tsp of balsamic vinegar

3 medium-sized potatoes, peeled and cubed

¼ tsp of black pepper, ground

½ tsp of Himalayan pink salt

Preparation:

Place the potatoes in a pot of boiling water and cook until fork-tender. Remove from the heat and transfer to serving plate. Sprinkle with some salt and set aside.

Preheat the oil in a large skillet over a medium-high temperature. Add garlic and stir-fry for about 3-4 minutes, or until translucent.

Add the meat chops and drizzle with vinegar. Sprinkle with some salt and pepper to taste and cook for about 5-7 minutes, stirring occasionally.

When the meat is golden brown, add tomatoes and onion. Cook until onions soften and translucent. Remove from the heat and serve with potatoes. Sprinkle all with fresh parsley and serve.

Nutritional information per serving: Kcal: 213, Protein: 21.6g, Carbs: 17g, Fats: 6.2g

31. Caribbean Beans

Ingredients:

2 cups of pink beans, soaked overnight

2 cups of vegetable broth

2 cups of water

1 large tomato

1 medium-sized red bell pepper, chopped

1 small onion, chopped

2 garlic cloves, minced

1 tsp of sea salt

¼ tsp of red pepper flakes

1 small plantain, peeled and chopped

Preparation:

Soak the beans overnight. Drain well and place in a pot of boiling water. Cook for 20 minutes, or until soften. Remove from the heat and drain well.

Now, place the beans in a heavy-bottomed pot and pour the vegetable broth. Bring it to a boil and add tomatoes, bell pepper, onion, garlic. Sprinkle with salt and pepper. Cook for 15 minutes more then add chopped plantain. Add water and bring it to a boil again. Reduce the simmer to low and cover with a lid. Cook for another 10 minutes and remove from the heat.

Serve warm.

Nutritional information per serving: Kcal: 59, Protein: 2.5g, Carbs: 12.4g, Fats: 0.6g

32. Winter Squash Soup

Ingredients:

8 oz. of butternut squash, chopped

1 cup of potatoes, cubed

1 small onion, chopped

1 cup of water

1 cup of vegetable broth

4 tbsp. of sour cream

1 garlic clove, minced

1 tsp of olive oil

1 tbsp. of fresh parsley, finely chopped

2 tbsp. of apple juice

½ tsp of salt

¼ tsp of black pepper, ground

Preparation:

Preheat the oil in a heavy-bottomed pot over a medium-high temperature. Add onion and stir-fry for about 3-4 minutes, or until translucent. Add the squash and potatoes.

Pour the vegetable broth, water, and apple juice. Stir well and bring it to a boil. Reduce the heat to low and cover with a lid. Cook for 40 minutes or until squash and potatoes soften.

Now, transfer all to the food processor and blend until creamy. Return to the pot and heat up. Sprinkle with some salt and pepper to taste. Remove from the heat and stir in the sour cream and parsley.

Serve warm.

Nutritional information per serving: Kcal: 108, Protein: 2.1g, Carbs: 19.5g, Fats: 2.9g

33. Pineapple Endive Smoothie

Ingredients:

¼ cup of pineapple chunks

½ cup of endive, chopped

1 cup of green grapes

1 large Granny Smith apple, cored

¼ cup of banana, sliced

1 cup of coconut milk

Preparation:

Wash and prepare the ingredients.

Now, combine pineapple, endive, grapes, apple, banana, and coconut milk in a food processor. Blend until nicely smooth and transfer to serving glasses.

Add few ice cubes and serve immediately.

Nutritional information per serving: Kcal: 394, Protein: 3.8g, Carbs: 37.4g, Fats: 29.1g

34. Creamy Salmon with Asparagus

Ingredients:

1 lb. of wild salmon fillets, cut into bite-sized pieces

2 cups of asparagus, trimmed and chopped

½ cup of sour cream

1 small onion, finely chopped

1 tbsp. of Dijon mustard

1 tbsp. of olive oil

1 tbsp. of apple cider vinegar

1 tsp of dried oregano, ground

½ tsp of salt

¼ tsp of black pepper, ground

1 tbsp. of fresh parsley, finely chopped

Preparation:

Wash the asparagus and trim off the woody ends. Cut into bite-sized pieces and transfer to a pot of boiling water. Cook until tender and remove from the heat. Drain and set aside.

Combine sour cream, vinegar, mustard, oregano, salt, pepper, and parsley in a mixing bowl. Stir well to mix and set aside.

Preheat the oil in a nonstick frying pan over a medium-high temperature. add onion and Sautee for about 3-4 minutes or until translucent.

Now, add salmon chops and cook for 3 minutes, stirring constantly. Add asparagus and pour the sour cream mixture. Cook for 3 minutes and remove from the heat.

Garnish with some lemon slices and serve immediately.

Nutritional information per serving: Kcal: 267, Protein: 24.8g, Carbs: 6.1g, Fats: 16.8g

35. Banana Quinoa Cereals

Ingredients:

1 cup of quinoa

2 cups of water

¼ cup of banana, chopped

1 cup of skim milk

¼ tsp of nutmeg, ground

1 tbsp. of honey

Preparation:

Combine quinoa and water in a deep pot. Bring it to a boil and then reduce the heat to low. Cover with a lid and cook for 15 minutes. Fluff the quinoa with a fork and let it cool for a while.

Transfer quinoa to a food processor and blend until creamy and smooth. Transfer to serving bowl and stir in the milk, nutmeg, honey, and cinnamon. Top with bananas or stir again. You can sprinkle with some chia seeds, but this is optional.

Serve immediately.

Nutritional information per serving: Kcal: 204, Protein: 8.1g, Carbs: 36.8g, Fats: 2.7g

36. Citrus Rice

Ingredients:

2 cups of white rice, long-grained

¼ cup of almonds, roughly chopped

½ cup of celery, chopped

1 tbsp. of olive oil

1 small onion, chopped

½ cup of orange juice, freshly squeezed

3 tbsp. of lemon juice, freshly squeezed

3 cups of water

¼ tsp of black pepper, ground

¼ tsp of Cayenne pepper, ground

½ tsp of sea salt

Preparation:

Place the rice in a deep pot. Add 3 cups of water and bring it to a boil. Cook for 10 minutes and remove from the heat. Drain well and set aside.

Preheat the oil in a large skillet over a medium-high temperature. Add onions and stir-fry for about 4-5 minutes, or until translucent. Add celery and cook for 5 minutes more.

Now, add orange juice, lemon juice, Cayenne pepper, and water. Bring it to a boil and stir in the rice. Reduce the heat to low and sprinkle with some salt. Cook for 2 minutes more. Remove from the heat and stir in the almonds. Let it stand for 5 minutes and serve.

Nutritional information per serving: Kcal: 286, Protein: 5.6g, Carbs: 53.9g, Fats: 4.8g

37. Oriental Turkey Skewers

Ingredients:

4 turkey breasts, skinless and boneless, cut into chunks

4 button mushrooms, stems removed

2 large onions, wedged

1 medium-sized orange, cut into quarters

1 large red bell pepper, roughly chopped

4 cherry tomatoes, whole

2 tbsp. of balsamic vinegar

4 tbsp. of olive oil

¼ tsp of ginger, ground

½ tsp of dried oregano, ground

½ tsp of salt

¼ tsp of black pepper, ground

4 skewers

Preparation:

Combine olive oil, vinegar, oregano, ginger, salt, and black pepper in a large bowl. Add the meat chunks and stir well to coat. Cover and marinate for 30 minutes in a refrigerator.

Now, thread the ingredients as follows: mushroom, turkey, onion, bell pepper, turkey, tomato. Repeat the process with the remaining ingredients and skewers.

Place the skewers in broiler about 6 inches from the heat source. Broil for 15 minutes on each side, brushing every 3 minutes with the remaining marinade.

Serve immediately.

Nutritional information per serving: Kcal: 150, Protein: 3.9g, Carbs: 14g, Fats: 9.8g

38. Shiitake Omelet

Ingredients:

5 large egg, beaten

1 small red onion, chopped

4 oz. of Shiitake mushrooms

1 garlic clove, crushed

1 tbsp. of fresh basil, finely chopped

2 tbsp. of skim milk

½ tsp of salt

¼ tsp of black pepper, ground

Preparation:

Preheat the oil in a large frying pan over a medium-high temperature. Add onion and stir-fry for about 3-4 minutes, or until translucent.

Add mushrooms and garlic and cook for 5 minutes, or until heated through.

Meanwhile, whisk the eggs with milk, salt, and pepper, in a mixing bowl. Pour the mixture into the pan and spread evenly with a wooden spatula. Sprinkle with basil and cook for 3-4 minutes, or until eggs are set. Scrap the bottom constantly to cook all evenly. Remove from the heat and serve immediately.

Nutritional information per serving: Kcal: 232, Protein: 17.7g, Carbs: 13.5g, Fats: 12.6g

39. Shrimps with Whole Wheat Pasta

Ingredients:

2 lbs. of large shrimps, cleaned and deveined

1 cup of whole wheat pasta

2 large bell peppers, chopped

½ large lemon, freshly juiced

4 tbsp. of olive oil

1 tsp of lemon zest

2 tbsp. of fresh parsley, finely chopped

½ tsp of salt

¼ tsp of black pepper, ground

Preparation:

Cook the pasta using package instructions. Remove from the heat and drain. Set aside.

Preheat the oil in a large frying pan over a medium-high temperature. Add garlic and cook for 1 minute. Add shrimps and sprinkle with some salt and pepper to taste. Cook for 2 minutes and then add bell pepper, lemon juice, and parsley. Cook for 5 minutes and then remove from the heat.

Stir into the pasta and sprinkle with lemon zest.

Serve immediately.

Nutritional information per serving: Kcal: 265, Protein: 30.5g, Carbs: 16.1g, Fats: 9.8g

40. Zucchini Cream Soup

Ingredients:

1 lb. of zucchinis, chopped

3 cups of vegetable broth

1 small onion, chopped

2 cups of milk, low-fat

4 tbsp. of Greek yogurt

1 tbsp. of pumpkin seeds

1 tsp of fresh sage, finely chopped

1 garlic clove, crushed

1 tsp of olive oil

½ tsp of salt

¼ tsp of black pepper, ground

Preparation:

Preheat the oil in a heavy-bottomed pot over a medium-high temperature. Add onion and garlic and stir-fry until translucent.

Now, add the zucchini chops and sprinkle with some sage to taste. Pour the vegetable broth and stir all well. Bring it to a boil and then reduce the heat to low. Cover with a lid and cook for about 25-30 minutes more. Remove from the heat and set aside to cool for a while.

Transfer all to the food processor and blend until creamy. Now, return to the pot and heat up. Sprinkle with salt and pepper and remove from the heat.

Stir in the Greek yogurt and milk. Garnish with some pumpkin seeds and serve immediately.

Nutritional information per serving: Kcal: 74, Protein: 5.5g, Carbs: 6.7g, Fats: 3.1g

41. Grilled Marinated Flank Steak

Ingredients:

2 lb. of flank steak

2 garlic cloves, minced

2 tbsp. of honey, raw

2 tbsp. of red wine vinegar

3 tbsp. of olive oil

1 tbsp. of ginger, freshly grated

½ tsp of salt

¼ tsp of black pepper, ground

Preparation:

Combine garlic, honey, vinegar, oil ginger, salt, and pepper in a large mixing bowl. Stir well to mix and then dip in the steaks. Cover with an aluminum boil or a lid and refrigerate for at least 2 hours.

Preheat grill to medium-high temperature. Place the steaks and grill for about 5-7 minutes on each side, or until desired doneness. Brush the steak constantly while grilling.

Remove from the heat and serve with steamed vegetables.

Nutritional information per serving: Kcal: 457, Protein: 50.7g, Carbs: 8.2g, Fats: 23.6g

42. Orange Quinoa Breakfast Porridge

Ingredients:

1 cup of white quinoa

1 cup of water

¼ cup of dried apricots, chopped

¼ cup of prunes, chopped

½ cup of orange juice

¼ tsp of cinnamon, ground

¼ cup of toasted almonds, roughly chopped

¼ tsp of ginger, ground

Preparation:

Combine quinoa and water in a pot and bring it to a boil. Reduce the heat to low and cook for about 10-15 minutes. Remove from the heat and fluff the quinoa with a fork. Set aside.

Now, combine cooked quinoa, apricots, and prunes. Drizzle with orange juice and sprinkle with ginger and cinnamon to taste. Stir all well and top with almonds before serving.

Enjoy!

Nutritional information per serving: Kcal: 314, Protein: 10.5g, Carbs: 53.1g, Fats: 7.6g

ADDITIONAL TITLES FROM THIS AUTHOR

70 Effective Meal Recipes to Prevent and Solve Being Overweight: Burn Fat Fast by Using Proper Dieting and Smart Nutrition

By Joe Correa CSN

48 Acne Solving Meal Recipes: The Fast and Natural Path to Fixing Your Acne Problems in Less Than 10 Days!

By Joe Correa CSN

41 Alzheimer's Preventing Meal Recipes: Reduce or Eliminate Your Alzheimer's Condition in 30 Days or Less!

By Joe Correa CSN

70 Effective Breast Cancer Meal Recipes: Prevent and Fight Breast Cancer with Smart Nutrition and Powerful Foods

By Joe Correa CSN

Made in the USA
Coppell, TX
10 February 2021